Essential Oils for Reducing Scars:
Best Essential Oils Recipes For Healing Fresh Scars And Reducing Old Scars

Table of content

Book introduction

Essential oils have been used for over thousands of years. They have been proven successful both in the scientific life as well as for amazing use in homes. Essential oils contain extractions from some useful plants, and from many parts of a plant. When essential oil was first discovered, the Egyptians and the Jews used to soak the plants in the oil and then used to take the oil by straining it.

Essential oils have amazing anti inflammation properties, protect against bacteria and they are very amazing anti oxidants. Essential oils can be used to serve numerous purposes such as window cleaners, fabric softeners, mosquito repellants, body washes, soaps, baby wipes, foot scrubs, as detergents, air refreshers and even in drinks, some of which are mentioned later in this book.

There are a few methods for the extraction of essential oils, namely distillation, expression, and solvent extraction. In the process of distillation, parts of the plants such as the leaves, flowers, stems barks and all are placed in the distillation can over water. As the water is steamed, the steam goes down the parts of the plant making the parts soft, extracting their oil and then the vapor passes through and is collected in the vessel. The vapor is cooled and condenses into liquid and that makes the essential oil.

In expression, the citrus fruits are used such as oranges and lemons. Their skins are peeled off and then used to make the essential oil. These essential oils of the citrus fruits are generally much cheaper than the other essential oils available. The process involved in the citrus fruits is somewhat similar to that of extracting the olive oil. They normally are expressed to get the essential oil or cold pressed which is similar to the extraction of olive oil.

An alternate process of extracting the essential oil apart from distillation is known as the solvent extraction. This process was found because some parts of the plant specially the flowers were found to be very delicate and lost their power when gone through the process of distillation because of the high heat in distillation. Apart from hexane, carbon dioxide is also used as a solvent in the extraction of essential oils.

Essential oils are widely used in pharmacies, and are considered to be of good use in medicines and for health purposes. They are also used in aromatherapy, which is for healing effects. They are also used to solve allergy conditions, irritated and itchy skin also.

Therefore, it can be seen that essential oils serve a wide variety of purposes and are really beneficial for human beings. They have a lot of natural ingredients in them and can be used in our day to lives. For your own benefit, it is a healthy choice to select a few essential oils and keep at your home for your use. You will find ahead 25 proven recipes of how essential oils can be used in your lives!

Recipe 01: Facewash for the sensitive skin

Description: In this eBook you will also find recipes of facewash which can be used on sensitive skins. Sensitive skins can be really painful, and itchy also. They can cause rashes on the skin making red patches which can be really painful. Below is a recipe of a foaming facewash for the sensitive skins.

Ingredients:

- Half teaspoon jojoba oil

- Ten drops of gentle baby essential oil
- Soap dispenser
- One teaspoon vitamin e oil
- Distilled water ¾ cup
- Two and half tablespoons of castile soap

Recipe:

- Take a dispenser and add in the water, the jojoba oil, the gentle baby essential oil, the vitamin e oil, the castile soap
- Mix all the ingredients together and stir well.
- Once they are stirred cover them with the pump and then use in your hand as required.
- Keep it away from the heat.

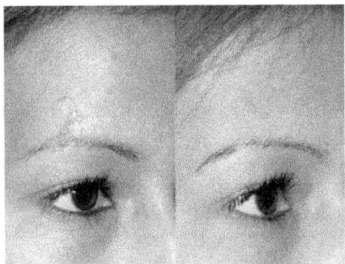

Recipe 02: Lavender cuticle oil
Description: This oil is specially made for skin purposes. For itchy skin, to keep the skin smooth and soft and so that it remains fresh all day. Besides it contains the apricot kernel oil which enhances its good properties. Below is the recipe of the lavender cuticle oil.

Ingredients:

- Half teaspoon of vitamin E oil

- One and half tablespoons of apricot kernel oil
- Twenty drops of lavender essential oil
- A dropper bottle

Recipe:

- Take the dropper bottle and put inside it the lavender essential oil, the apricot kernel oil and the vitamin e oil.
- Combine all ingredients and shake it well.
- Swirl the bottle to combine. Once done, whenever you have to use it put on your skin through the dropper once you have washed and dried your skin.
- Rub and massage your skin until the oil in it has been absorbed.
- Whenever skin becomes dry you can use it.
- Store it in a cool place.

Recipe 03: Peppermint foot scrub

Description: When walking barefoot the skin on our feet becomes dry, and starts to wear off. This problem becomes severe in the winter season because of the dry season. This peppermint foot scrub contains vital ingredients to keep the feet smooth and moist and prevent dryness. The avocado oil in this scrub is a nice emollient which prevents dryness of the skin.

Ingredients;

- ¼ cup of baking soda
- ¼ cup of sugar
- Ten drops of peppermint essential oil
- A glass jar
- ¼ cup of avocado oil

Recipe:

- Take the glass jar and pour in the peppermint essential oil and the avocado oil.

- Then add in the dry ingredients that's the baking soda and the sugar.
- Stir well to combine all ingredients.
- Keep applying the scrub on your foot and notice the change in your skin and its silkiness!

Recipe 04: Homemade moisturizing vanilla lip balm

Description: Winters bring along dryness along with them, and our lips start to become red and dry. They start to stretch with dryness and it is necessary to keep them moist. Lip balms are widely used for this purpose. Below is such a recipe of a homemade vanilla flavored lip balm to serve this purpose and to keep the lips moist.

Ingredients:

- One drop of geranium essential oil
- Two drops of bergamot essential oil
- Two drops of vanilla extract
- One gram of vitamin E oil
- Three grams of coconut oil
- Five grams of beeswax
- Five grams of shea butter
- Seven grams of avocado oil

Recipe:

- Take a double boiler and put in it the coconut oil, the vitamin e oil, the beeswax, shea butter, avocado oil, and the vanilla extract.
- Stir it until everything is mixed and melted and remove it from heat and now add in the geranium essential oil and the bergamot essential oil.
- Pour it into lipstick shape tubes and let it cool and let it set.

Recipe 05: Aloe vera soothing sun spray

Description: Aloe vera has many benefits to the skin and can be used for a variety of purposes. Aloe vera lets the skin recover really fast after any kind of itching problems. It heals the itchy and irritated skin. It acts as a great anti oxidant and keeps the skin really smooth and nice to touch. Below is a recipe of an aloe vera spray which you can make at your home.

Ingredients:

- ¾ cup of aloe vera gel
- Ten drops of peppermint essential oil
- Ten drops of lavender essential oil
- One tablespoon of coconut oil
- One cup of water
- A spray bottle

Recipe:

- Take the spray bottle and add in the water, the alovera gel, the peppermint essential oil, the lavender essential oil, and the coconut oil.
- Stir and mix the bottle until all the ingredients are properly mixed and stirred.
- Close the bottle and use it for spraying on the skin for a smooth and ravishing effect.

Recipe 06: Emergency burn compress or wash

Description: A burn on our skins can be very painful and difficult to handle. This recipe of essential oil burn compress provides quick relief from burns. Below is the recipe of it.

Ingredients:

- One pint of water at a temperature of 50 degrees Fahrenheit
- Five drops of lavender oil

Recipe:

- Add the lavender oil in to the water as to properly mix in the oil with water.
- With a help of a soft cloth or towel dip the cloth in to the liquid and let it soak for about 10 minutes.
- Put the cloth on the burnt area for a while and then remove.
- You can also soak the burnt area in the oil to get relief.

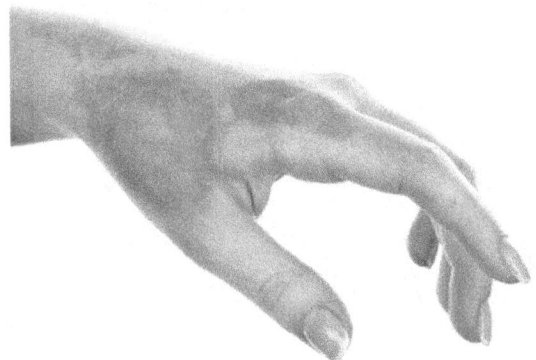

Recipe 07: After burn essential oil formula

Description: Instead of using the tubes available in the market at such expensive rates it is better to apply essential oil to the burnt area. Here we provide you with a recipe of essential oil for the treatment of burns.

Ingredients:

- Two drops of peppermint essential oil
- 25 drops of lavender essential oil
- Two ounces of sunflower oil

Recipe:

- Mix in the peppermint essential oil, the lavender essential oil and the sunflower oil.
- Mix all the oils and then apply on the affected area two to three times a day.
- It will cure in no time.

Recipe 08: Homemade burn formula

Description: This recipe of essential oil is very easy and quick to make at home. It is recommended to make it and store it to use in emergency conditions. Below is the recipe of it.

Ingredients:

- Eight drops of lavender essential oil or five drops of roman chamomile oil
- One bowl of cold water

Recipe:

- Mix the cold water and the lavender or chamomile oil until the oil is properly diffused with the water.
- You can add ice cubes to make the water colder.
- Dip the burnt area in to this oil for immense relief.
- You can also take a cloth, dip in the oil and then apply the cloth on to your burnt skin.

Recipe 09: Essential oil blend for sun burns

Description: People go out on the beach to enjoy and to relax. Sometimes the heat of the sun is so severe that instead of getting a tan we get sun burns which are very irritating and sometimes very painful as well. Below you will find a recipe of a comforting blend to cure sun burns.

Ingredients:

- One tub of cool water
- One drop of pepper mint
- Two drops of helichrysum
- two drops of roman chamomile
- eight drops of lavender essential oil

Recipe:

- In a tub of cool water, add in the pepper mint, helichrysum, roman chamomile and the lavender essential oil and mix.
- Apply this mixture on to the affected sunburn and let it soak for about 15 minutes.
- Do this twice or thrice a day to get complete relief.

Recipe 10: Soothing blend to cure burns

Description: This essential oil is to cure and sooth the burns on the skin which cause real pain. It is fairly easy and quick to make with only a few ingredients. Below is the recipe of it.

Ingredients:

- twenty drops of lavender essential oil
- five teaspoons of fresh aloe vera juice
- one teaspoon of sea buckthorn oil

Recipe:

- Take a glass container of one ounce and add in the lavender essential oil, aloe vera juice and the sea buckthorn oil and mix.
- Before using shake the bottle and with the help of a cotton ball apply the oil very gently and carefully to the affected area.

Recipe 11: Essential oil recipe to mend scars

Description: This recipe of essential oil is made to mend scars on the skin. Sometimes the scars on the skin can cause real irritation and problems. For this we have provided you with a recipe of essential oil. Below is the recipe of it.

Ingredients:

- two ounces of grape seed oil
- five drops of tea tree oil

- five drops of lavender oil

Recipe:

- Take a glass container and add in the grape seed oil, the tea tree oil and the lavender oil and mix properly.
- Let sit the oil for a day or two before applying it on your scars.
- Apply twice a day.

Recipe 12: Anti-aging carrot seed oil serum

Description: Carrot seed essential oil is considered to be the best essential oil that is used to the treatment of scars. They heal the scars and reduce them. Carrot seed essential oil is used in most scar treatments and here is another recipe which uses carrot seed essential oil.

In this recipe, carrot seed essential oil is used to make an anti aging serum for the treatment of scars.

Ingredients:

- Prickly pear oil- 1 tablespoon
- Argan oil- 2 teaspoon
- Carrot seed oil- 5 drops
- Lavender oil- 3 drops
- Frankincense oil-2 drops
- A small funnel
- Amber dropper bottle of 2 oz

Recipe:

- Use a small funnel to pour in the prickly pear oil and the argan oil in the amber dropper bottle.
- Now add in the carrot seed oil, lavender oil and the frankincense oil.
- Close the bottle and shake to mix in all the ingredients.

- To use, put in 2 to 3 drops on the palm of your hand and apply on your face or where the scars are most visible.
- This essential oil can also be applied when you are under makeup.

Recipe 13: Skin lightening cream to remove scars

Description: The carrot seed essential oil contains high amounts of antioxidants which help the body to recover from any damage it might have went through. Quite simply it can be said that carrot seed essential oil has the properties of being a healing agent.

In this recipe, carrot seed essential oil is used as a skin lightening cream which you can apply on your face and if you have some scars or burns these will then go away by the use of this cream. The shea butter added gives softness to the skin and a nice fragrance to the cream as well.

Ingredients:

- Shea butter- 1 tablespoon
- Carrot seed essential oil- 2 drops
- Lemon oil- 2 drops
- Frankincense oil- 2 drops

Recipe:

- Take a bottle and add in the shea butter and the carrot seed essential oil.
- Mix properly to mix both the ingredients.
- Now add in the lemon oil and the frankincense oil and shake to mix all the ingredients together.
- Use this cream in little quantities and apply on your face every night before sleeping to avail its benefits.

Recipe 14: Carrot seed essential oil facial mask for the treatment of scars

Description: The following carrot seed essential oil recipe is of a rejuvenating facial mask which will help you in the treatment of your scars. It might take some time to heal the scars you have but carrot seed essential oil is an excellent remedy in the treatment of scars and burns.

You can use the following recipe to get rid of all kinds of scars you have. You should however keep in mind that it will take a long time in the treatment of scars and it depends upon how intensive the scar is.

Ingredients:

- Bentonite clay- 1 teaspoon
- Aloe vera gel- 1 teaspoon
- Carrot seed essential oil- 2 to 3 drops
- A small bowl
- A spoon
- A face mask brush

Recipe:

- In a bowl, mix in the bentonite clay and the aloe vera gel by the spoon
- Now add in the carrot seed essential oil drops and mix.
- With the help of a face mask brush apply this facial mask on your face and particularly where the scars are most prominent.
- Rinse your face with warm water.
- You will see the results instantly.

Recipe 15: Sun damaged skin soother

Description: There might be times when you might have gone to the beach and in the water and it would have caused your skin to be really itchy and scars might have appeared.

Itching the rashes and scars can make the matter more worse and the scars can deepen. Apart from that, the sand or sea creatures might bite you thereby giving you some scar or a bruise. It will be better in that case to apply this sun damaged skin soother instead of a chemically stuffed cream from the supermarket.

Ingredients:

- Carrot seed essential oil- 5 drops
- Aloe vera gel- ¼ cup
- Amber glass jar- 4 oz

Recipe:

- In your amber glass jar add in the carrot seed essential oil drops.
- Now add the aloe vera gel and mix properly.
- Put this mixture on your affected skin area or the burns or scars.
- Let it be applied for a while before washing.
- Give it some time to heal the scar before washing away the soothing cream.

Recipe 16: Scar healing serum recipe

Description: This serum is used to heal the scars one might have on their body or on their face. Scars can look really bad specially if they are on the face and this serum recipe is an excellent one in order to heal the scars.

In this recipe of the serum, a variety of essential oils are used all of which have excellent healing properties for scars. Follow this recipe in order to get rid of the scars.

Ingredients:

- Roll on bottle- 1
- Funnel- 1
- Castor oil- 1/3 cup
- Tamanu oil- 2 tablespoon
- Lavender essential oil- 5 drops

- Helichrysum essential oil- 5 drops
- Carrot seed essential oil- 5 drops
- Elemi essential oil- 5 drops
- Frankincense essential oil-5 drops

Recipe:

- Take the roll on bottle and add in the castor oil and the tamanu oil.
- Now add in the lavender essential oil, helichrysum essential oil, carrot seed essential oil, elemi essential oil and the frankincense essential oil.
- Add all of these essential oils through the funnel to avoid mess.
- Cap the bottle tightly and then shake properly to let all the essential oils mix together.
- Apply this serum on the affected areas atleast twice a day as it will give the best results.
- You can even apply it three times a day if you wish for quick results.
- Keep on applying this serum to get rid of scars.

Recipe 17: Gentle oil blend for reducing scars

Description: The following recipe is of an oil blend made in order to reduce the scars you might have on your face. This gentle oil blend will work best on you if you have a sensitive skin so you need not worry about your scars.

The important thing to remember is to mix in the carrier oil blends gently which will work best in the removal of scars. Carrier oil should be blended properly in this recipe provided you have a very sensitive skin.

Ingredients:

- Rosehip seed oil- 1 tablespoon
- Calendula oil- 1 tablespoon

- Tamanu oil- 1 tablespoon

Recipe:

- In a bottle, add in the rosehip seed oil, calendula oil and the tamanu oil.
- Mix to blend in all the oils properly.
- Gently apply this oil with your fingers on your face.
- Dab your face with a paper towel in order to remove the excess oil.
- Let it stay for a while before washing with water to provide quick result.

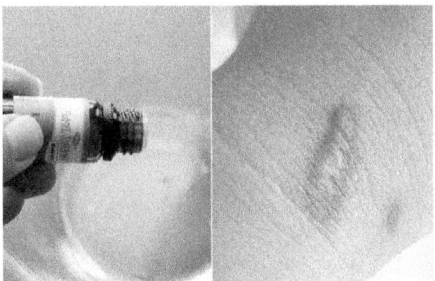

Recipe 18: Strong oil blend for reducing scars

Description: This oil blend might be a little expensive to buy as both the rosehip essential oil and the helichrysum essential oil are quite expensive. The results however, are very affective and your scars will be healed in no time.

This oil blend provides the perfect solution for your skin without the need for any moisturizers or other useless skin care products. This recipe contains a citrus oil, it will be best to use this oil blend on your face in the night time in order to protect your skin from getting damaged by the sun.

Ingredients:

- Rosehip seed oil- half cup

- Helichrysum essential oil- 15 drops
- Mandarin oil- 15 drops
- Tea tree oil- 10 drops

Recipe:

- In a bottle, add in the rosehip seed oil.
- Now add in the helichrysum essential oil.
- Add in the mandarin oil and finally the tea tree oil.
- Cap the bottle tightly.
- Mix properly and make sure that all the oils are blended in perfectly.
- Apply this oil blend as a moisturizer on your face and let it stay for a while without washing for quick results.
- You can apply it twice all through the night.

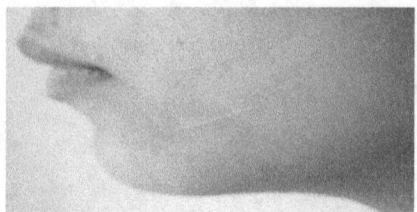

Recipe 19: Clean wounds and scars

Description: There is always a likely chance of you getting a scar or a wound if you go on a picnic. While some wounds disappear themselves some chose to be stubborn and develop in to life long scars. The following recipe teaches you how to clean your wounds and prevent them in to developing in to scars in the easiest way possible.

Lemon is a natural antiseptic which is used in the treatment of burns, wounds and scars. Lemon prevents infection from developing.

Ingredients:

- Beeswax pellets- ¼ cup
- Coconut oil- ¾ cup
- Lemon oil- 12 drops
- Lavender essential oil- 12 drops
- Tea tree oil- 12 drops

Recipe:

- In a double boiler add the beeswax pellets and the coconut oil and melt both of them on low heat until both incorporate together.
- The beeswax might take a longer time to melt.
- Remove from heat and let it cool.
- Now add in the lemon oil and the lavender essential oil and mix.
- Finally add in the tea tree oil and mix all the ingredients.
- Pour this mixture in to a bottle.
- Apply to affected areas and dab with a paper towel to remove the excess oil.
- Apply twice or thrice a day for quick results.

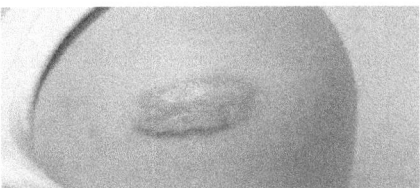

Recipe 20: Scar removal salve

Description: This recipe is for the fresh scars and it is great in healing them. It has a longer staying power than the healing oil and will heal your scars much quickly. The lavender essential oil added gives a nice fragrance to this oil and is nice for your skin as well.

The shea butter gives a smooth texture to your skin and an amazing fragrance as well. The beeswax may take a longer time to melt in properly. You can use this recipe whenever you get a fresh scar and use it to remove the scars completely.

Ingredients:

- Beeswax- 3 tablespoons
- Shea butter- 2 tablespoons
- Hemp seed oil- 1 tablespoon
- Vitamin E oil- 1 tablespoon
- Lavender essential oil- 5 drops

Recipe:

- In a double boiler, melt in the beeswax and the shea butter.
- The shea butter might take a long time to melt.
- Remove from heat once the beeswax and the shea butter are melted and incorporated together.
- Now add in the hemp seed oil and the vitamin E oil.
- Finally add in the lavender essential oil.
- Mix together all the ingredients.
- Pour the mixture in to little salve tins and let them harden before use.
- You can use this salve on stretch marks to scars and the vitamin E oil added works best for healing scars.
- Use this oil twice a day for best results.

Recipe 21: Simple healing oil for scars

Description: This healing oil is great for new scars that still stitch together and have not opened. All you need for this healing oil is just 2 ingredients and need to apply it to heal your fresh scars. The DMAE is a natural amino acid which repairs the skin and nourishes it at the same time.

Using this healing oil, you will notice the results almost instantly.

Ingredients:

- Grape seed essential oil- ¼ cup
- DMAE (Dimenthylaminoethanol) -5 drops
- Dropper bottle

Recipe:

- In the dropper bottle, combine the grape seed essential oil and the DMAE.
- Cap the bottle and shake it to mix both the ingredients.
- Use 2 or 3 drops on your scar or more depending upon how large is your scar.
- Apply it twice or thrice a day.

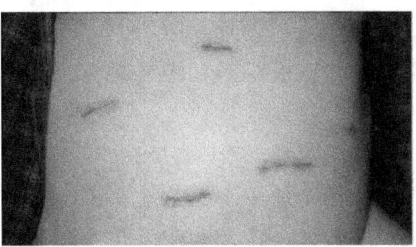

Recipe 22: Anti scar blend

Description: The following recipe is for a 10 percent dilution made for those who have old scars and wish to reduce them. For newer scars, you need a 5 percent dilution. The ingredients used in this recipe might be a bit expensive but they are very affective and can heal your oldest scars.

Ingredients:

- A 20-ml roller bottle
- Helichrysum essential oil- 16 drops
- Frankincense essential oil- 16 drops

- Geranium essential oil- 8 drops
- Tamanu oil- 1/3 bottle

Recipe:

- Fill 1/3 of the bottle with tamanu oil.
- Now add in the helichrysum essential oil, geranium essential oil and the frankincense essential oil.
- Cap the bottle tightly and shake to mix in all the ingredients properly.
- Apply to your scar 2 to 3 times daily for best and quick results.

Recipe 23: Scar smoothening and brightening skin recipe

Description: Fruits and vegetables have excellent capability to heal all kinds of scars and they have excellent healing properties as well. This recipe is fast and simple for those scars that are fresh and wounds that have healed but their presence is still there.

Ingredients:

- Garden fresh tomato or a juice of 1 lemon
- Cotton ball- 1

Recipe:

- Juice either the lemon or the garden tomato in a bowl.
- Soak the cotton ball in the lemon juice.
- Now when the cotton ball has completely soaked in the lemon juice dab the cotton ball on your charred skin where there are scars.
- Let the juice soak in to your scars to let them heal.
- Let it dry and do not wash till the morning.
- Wash the next morning and see the effects.

Recipe 24: Essential oil using apricot oil

Description: You can use as many of the essential oils you desire in this recipe. This recipe uses a combination of many kinds of essential oils which is why it is very effective in the healing of your scars.

Though it may seem expensive to buy all the essential oils but once you are done with its making this recipe will work wonders for your scarred skin. They will heal and give you good and quick results.

Ingredients:

- Rosehip oil- 1 oz
- Apricot kernel oil- 1 oz
- Helichrysum essential oil- 5 drops
- Carrot seed essential oil- 5 drops
- Frankincense essential oil- 5 drops
- Calendula oil- 5 drops
- Rosemary essential oil- 5 drops
- Lavender essential oil- 10 drops

Recipe:

- In a bottle, add the rosehip oil, apricot kernel oil, helichrysum essential oil, carrot seed oil, frankincense oil, calendula oil, rosemary oil and the lavender essential oil.
- Cap the bottle and mix it to combine all the ingredients.
- Apply it to your scar twice daily for quick results.

Recipe 25: Acne serum to remove acne scars

Description: During your teens you might get a lot of acne on your face which are considered to be the one of the signs of puberty. While the acne goes away as you reach the age of 18 and above some acne might leave scars.

Ingredients:

- Lavender essential oil- 8 drops
- Tea tree essential oil- 15 drops
- Geranium essential oil- 2 drops
- Patchouli essential oil- 3 drops
- Grapefruit essential oil- 3 drops
- Tamanu oil- ½ teaspoon
- Grapeseed oil- 4 tablespoons

Recipe:

- Add in the tamanu oil in your bottle first.
- Now add in the lavender essential oil, tea tree essential oil, geranium essential oil, patchouli essential oil, grapefruit oil and the grape seed oil and mix properly.
- Massage on to your skin every day for a smooth and scar free skin.

Conclusion

At the end of this e book, first I would like to thank all the readers, who took out their time and downloaded this ebook. I am particularly thankful to all the readers out there. The advantages of essential oils have long been known, and to study them and the ingredients and the recipes which can be made using these essential oils can help you a great deal in your life.

This ebook contains 25 valid and authentic recipes using essential oils as their core ingredient. Essential oils can be used to treat headaches, migraines, cold, congestion, flu, mental tiredness, sleep problems, anxiety problems, for calming babies and many many more.

This ebook however explains in full detail about how to use essential oils for the treatment of scars and how to heal them.

By downloading this ebook you can make sure that your life will be at a much better pace then it was ever before. Essential oils have a lot of advantages and the biggest advantage this has is that it is much better to use these essential oil recipes which are natural rather than using tablets and medicines and tubes from the market which are not only harmful for the health but also uselessly expensive.

Following this ebook you can get 25 fool proof recipes about how to use essential oils for the treatment of scars.

I hope that all of you had an amazing time reading this ebook and would appreciate your comments on this ebook. Feel free to ask any question or query you wish to ask. In the end I would like to wish each and every reader a happy reading! Adios!

FREE Bonus Reminder

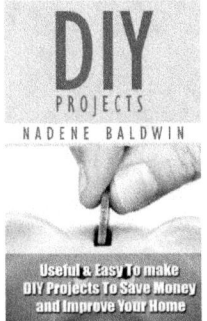

If you have not grabbed it yet, please go ahead and download your special bonus report *"DIY Projects. 13 Useful & Easy To Make DIY Projects To Save Money & Improve Your Home!"*

Simply Click the Button Below

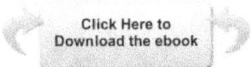

OR **Go to This Page**

http://diyhomecraft.com/free

BONUS #2: More Free & Discounted Books or Products

Do you want to receive more Free/Discounted Books or Products?

We have a mailing list where we send out our new Books or Products when they go free or with a discount on Amazon. Click on the link below to sign up for Free & Discount Book & Product Promotions.

=> Sign Up for Free & Discount Book & Product Promotions <=

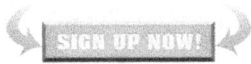

OR Go to this URL

http://zbit.ly/1WBb1Ek